Praise for *Dancing with Breast Cancer*

The poet Muriel Rukeyser once said, "What would happen if one woman told the truth about her life? The world would split open." In *Dancing with Breast Cancer*, Janay Cosner tells the truth about her life as a breast cancer patient and survivor: her story of fear and pain and loss but also, ultimately, her story of a path to new self knowledge. Cosner calls each poem "a snapshot" of her journey, and indeed these poems offer vivid images of the journey from breast cancer diagnosis to treatment to remission. What does it mean to be a survivor, these poems ask. What does it mean to be a warrior? "Come dance with me," Cosner invites the reader, and we do as we follow her amazing journey and self-transformation.

icole Cooley,
hor of *Breach*

Janay Cosner writes about her personal odyssey with breast cancer in a way that makes it our journey as well. The emotions are the doorway as we engage with the anger, the doubt, the fear of the unknown, the specter of change, and, yes, the wry humor that lives with Janay and with us along this often lonely path. Her language is direct and engaging, her images rock solid, and the attitude that permeates this body of work—like Janay herself—is unyielding.

—Craig Sipe,
author of *Hero Sandwich*

"Dear Girls"—I *so love* this love letter of solidarity to women everywhere, whose final break-neck turn (forgive me for not wanting to steal the poem's thunder by telling it here!) once heard, will be immediately seared into memory and, if such a thing were possible, it should be tattooed—irrespective of gender—onto every living creature with a breast bone!

—Rick Hilles,
author of *Map of the Lost World*

Dancing with Breast Cancer is Janay Cosner's entry to a debutante ball no one wants to attend. And yet, here is form for fear. Language for pain. In a ballet, in the improvised steps of hip-hop or funk, her poems dance across the page even when the body resists. Some of us will read from safe, for now, armchairs, while others will recognize themselves. All must laugh and cry and finally cheer her final line, "Come dance with me."

—Mary McLaughlin Slechta,
author of *Wreckage on a Watery Moon*

Janay Cosner's *Dancing with Breast Cancer* documents the speaker's changing perception of her past, her body, the world, and her life. Through keen imagery and with wisdom, honesty, and humor, these poems do what poetry does best: they teach us to understand. Cosner writes, "The outside world/ comes to me." Indeed, we have come to her to listen, but we also close this book changed, "out of breath and glorious."

—Robert Ostrom,
author of *The Youngest Butcher in Illinois*

DANCING WITH BREAST CANCER

A Memoir in Poems

JANAY COSNER

*This book is dedicated to
my husband, Richard—
my rock.*

CONTENTS

INTRODUCTION

One out of eight women is diagnosed with breast cancer. Shocked, panicked, angry, depressed, and overwhelmed are only a few of the emotions I experienced when I was diagnosed. This book, *Dancing with Breast Cancer*, presents my personal odyssey and takes readers from the discovery of cancer through surgery, chemo, and radiation treatments and then finally to my "new normal."

Each poem in this memoir is a snapshot of my journey: some are pretty, some ugly, some humorous, but all are sprinkled with attitude. A pen and paper were a great comfort to me in the middle of the night, at doctors' appointments, and in many other stressful situations. Writing about my experiences let me process my emotions and led to insights that helped me surmount difficult obstacles.

Dancing also helped me deal with the traumatic events of breast cancer. I was born a dancer and loved to move my body. I felt free; I was flying. Soon after my diagnosis, I had to learn a new kind of dance, the dance with doctors and cancer. My cancer dance spun me in circles. I watched as my body lost muscle tone. The mutilations and baldness lowered my self-esteem, and my body image suffered. I became too weak to dance. My only dance then was my dance with words—poetry. It was not easy to catch the beat of who I would become. After many difficult months, I came back stronger, and my new dance of life began.

At readings of *Dancing with Breast Cancer*, one survivor told me she felt many of the feelings experienced in the poems but never said them out loud. A husband of a breast cancer survivor cried, saying he never realized what his wife went through. An oncologist was surprised, saying, "My patients never expressed these feelings to my face." We all know someone who has had breast cancer, but do we know how it feels to go through this life-changing event? I have written *Dancing with Breast Cancer* in the clearest language possible so that it can be accessible to breast cancer patients, survivors, family members, caretakers, doctors, nurses, medical centers, support groups, and book clubs.

This book is for all the women I've never met who have or had breast cancer. I cried, screamed, unzipped myself, and spilled my guts to create the poems in this book. I hope my observations will help people not only to understand that breast cancer changes lives forever but also to recognize that in this change, powerful lessons can be learned: Don't sweat the small stuff. Live each day fully. You are stronger than you think. Dance fast and furious.

We dance for laughter,
we dance for tears,
we dance for madness,
we dance for fears,
we dance for screams,
we are the dancers,
we create the dreams.

—Albert Einstein

PART I
DIAGNOSIS AND SURGERY

Life is not about waiting for the storm to pass.
It's about learning to dance in the rain.

—Vivian Greene

Mammo (Oh No!) Gram

The cold diagnostic machine squeezes
my flattened breasts like two fried eggs
and finds a suspicious abnormality in the left.

Close the blinds,
see only what I want to see.

Ultrasound follows.
Like a glazed doughnut,
gooey salve slathered on my breast.
The wand lights up at six o'clock,
disco lights, but no party.

Close the blinds.

Biopsy is like a turkey baster run in reverse.
Click! Clack! The needle sucks out tissue.
Trussed like a bird,
I teeter out of the office.

Close the blinds.

Three days later, a tumor found,
the size of a blueberry.

Close the blinds.

I Knew, I Didn't Know

Friday, a biopsy wand flares.
Saturday, a whirl around the dance floor
at Pam and Joe's wedding.

The bandaged breast binds. Sunday,
I cook fajitas for friends,
run the dishwasher.

Monday, in a hushed voice,
looking at my doctor husband, the radiologist
rattles off words about a positive biopsy.

I am a wilting wallflower in the room
as they discuss appointments—
a PET scan, blood tests, x-rays.

The dance of illness begins,
my new partner, cancer.

Ballerina

I am going on vacation to the sick world.
No lounge chairs or pink drinks with umbrellas,
no pulsating Caribbean drums, no perfect white beaches,

just gray doctors' offices full of health magazines and steel chairs.

My days full of biopsies, x-rays, PET scans, thumping MRIs,
pink, yellow, green pills.

I bond with patients:
> *What are you in for?*
> *What stage?*
> *How many treatments to go?*
> *You look great.*

No longer the daring bikini-clad blonde,
I am terrified, twirling off balance on tiptoes.

I want to go home.

How Do I Tell My Children?

(The doctor said breast cancer would
take a year out of my life.)

Circle one.

A. Yell "Timber" and run like hell.

B. Lie and tell them I am going on a trip around the world.

C. Don't ever tell them.

D. Say that I am going to a fat farm.

E. Underestimate the seriousness of the diagnosis.

F. Tell the truth.

G. None of the above.

So Many Doctor Appointments

Another cold office,
another steel chair,
I want to slip to the tile,
like Gumby every time.

Peel me off the floor.

The Sounds of Cancer in the Examining Room

Heavy footsteps of Nunn Bush loafers in the hall,
sharp clip-clop of high heels,
rustle and rattle of health magazines,
the crackling of paper on the examining table.
Doors open and close sadly.
An angry air conditioner blows.
A sink pours out someone's tears.
Hard chairs creak with worry,
muted murmurs of concern,

the howl of the lone wolf,
me.

Conversation Heart Cereal Treats

Makes 10 bars

2 tablespoons butter
20 large marshmallows
3 cups frosted cat cereal with marshmallow bits
10 large conversation heart candies

Preparation
Mix ingredients, except for the hearts, together and press in pan.
Bake at 350° for 40 minutes.

Press heart candies on top of the treats. One heart per bar.
Apply these "right-on" sayings for doctors.

> PLEASE TAKE CARE OF ME.
>
> PUT YOURSELF IN MY BRA.
>
> PLEASE TAKE TIME WITH ME.
>
> UNDERSTAND MY PANIC.
>
> PLEASE DON'T TREAT ME LIKE EVERYONE ELSE.
>
> GIVE ME HOPE.
>
> PLEASE BE WITH ME EVERY STEP OF THE WAY.
>
> DON'T LET THIS BE ANOTHER DAY IN THE OFFICE.
>
> PLEASE TELL ME I WON'T DIE.
>
> UNDERSTAND HOW MY WORLD IS IMPLODING.

Dear Girls,

(Before lumpectomy or mastectomy decision)
I knew you had power
in tenth-grade bonehead geometry
when the guys took their problems
up to Mr. Square's desk to get
a better look at you, muttering
Great rack! under their breaths.

Later you ballooned into 36Ds.
Men brought Beluga caviar in Las Vegas.
Sugar daddies showered you
with Chanel No. 5,
a ruby necklace to accent your allure.
You swayed through the ages—
rock-n-roll, disco, and hip-hop
in low-cut sweaters,
push-up and plunge bras,
two beautiful milky mountains.

We were best buds,
but now you're sick.
We have to break up.
I need space.
I'm sorry, but I need to keep
my options open.
Anyway, I think I loved you more
than you loved me,
but I will never forget you.

Sadly,
Janay

Arrested Development

(Before lumpectomy or mastectomy decision)
I had a dream.
I'm ten again—my ponytail swirls,
I play with paper dolls,
hopscotch on the driveway,
dance to Ricky Nelson on vinyl.
I'm the perfect Barbie doll.

My body looks ten again,
hairless and breastless.
I'm married to the perfect Ken,
my paper dolls my two children.
I hopscotch to Europe and the Caribbean,
dance to Pitbull on CDs.

Now the nightmare begins.

I'm Not Proud of Myself

I am a tsunami,
kick dents in wastebaskets,
throw a bag of cheese at a truck,
scream at nurses,
cancel my surgery,
fire my chemo doctor.
I want to say I'm sorry.
My anger is misplaced.

Having cancer is like driving a bus without steering,
and my feet can't reach the brakes.

Lumpectomy

"The idea of waiting for something
makes it more exciting."
But Andy Warhol
didn't have breast cancer.

The Therapist

Dressed in tweed,
she looked professional.

In her pink office,
I perch on a plush flowered chair,

my grandmother's hanky
balled in my fist.

She listens. I want to rant
but don't have the energy.

I feel like an anemone that would fold
at the first question. She writes

key phrases in a soft-covered book.
I say, *I'm shrinking! I'm scared*

of surgery, chemo, and radiation.
She says one thing that makes sense.

You're used to being in control of your life,
but now you're not.

Syncopated Surgery

aches, agony, bed rails, beeps, biopsies, LOSS, PAIN, LOSS, blood, bloodstained, blur, breathing tube, bright Chihuly lights, carve, cold room, cut up, cut to pieces, damage, deceased brother yelling in the distance, deform, destroy, LOSS, PAIN, LOSS, disfigurement, dizzy, doctors, family waving on the ceiling, LOSS, PAIN, finger clip, gas, gash, gauze, grief, gurney, hack, havoc, heartache, heartbeat, heartbreaking, hiss of oxygen, incomplete inflamed, invasion, IV, lacerate, lime green gown, maim, mangle, LOSS, mar, mask, metallic snip of shears, morphine, mourning, mutilation, LOSS, PAIN, LOSS, needles, nurses, ordeal, oxygen mask, paper slippers, pillage, pills, pulverize, rattling rainsticks turned upside down, ravage, recovery room, rend, rip, sad, scalpel, scars, PAIN, sedation, shatter, sterile, stitches, swoosh, tears, theater, throb, torture, tubes, whispered prayers, woe, zero-to-ten pain scale

New Position

After surgery I stand
when I vomit.
I refuse to get on my knees.
That would mean cancer has won.

Pain pills

turn me into a scary person.
I am in slow motion,
no makeup,
chipped nail polish,
straggly uncombed hair,
the same nightgown every day,
a bath if I have the strength.

Who am I?
I used to wear makeup to the gym,
used to flaunt Naples blue nail polish
on my filed fingernails,
used to comb coiffed hair in place,
used to wear satiny night clothes,
used to relax in a mile-high bubble bath.

I am afraid of this stranger,
afraid of being her.

Vicodin

We had an addictive affair
after a hysterectomy in '03.
I, your hot-girl mistress. You, my bad-boy painkiller.
We drifted in underwater euphoria.
I remember a tough breakup.

Today after surgery I relapsed,
our dalliance difficult to control.
I am lightheaded, dizzy.
You pull me away from pain's grip.
With you, I can disappear.

Vicodin, you were there
when I needed you in the sorrow of my lost
womanhood years ago. Now in my disfigurement,
you make life easier by obscuring it.
But soon I must cut you off.

I need to reappear,
come up from underwater.
I'm swimming away, towing a small victory.

Night Fears after Surgery

2:30 a.m.
   Cancer ghosts flap near the curtains.

The radiation rat scratches
   dust balls under the bed.

The chemo cat howls
   to be let in.

I wish I were a doll,
   my face frozen,

my body free of pain,
   so a young girl would cuddle me,

wrap me in a blanket,
   take away the night terrors,

like when I was a child,
   my eyes tired from crying.

Christmas Cancer

Santa rides at the end of the Macy's parade.
I wonder what he will bring me this year—

maybe eyebrows with stencils and glue,
or surgery corsets with bra cups,

crisp blouses with pockets inside
for easy access to surgical drains,

stylish beanies, turbans with bangs,
baseball caps with polyester hair,

chemo hats with crazy sayings:
"I'm Having a No Hair Day,"

"Bald Chicks Rock,"
"My Oncologist Does My Hair."

Maybe I'll ask him
for a lump of coal instead.

Fa La La

I binge on Christmas movies
on the Lifetime and Hallmark channels.
I'm in a fantasy world,

where it snows in LA,
where a workaholic boyfriend
two-times the heroine

but all is made right when she
wishes on a Christmas star.
Where is that star now?

Only 14 more shopping days until chemo.
Where is that miracle?

You'll Be Fine

What will people tell me today?

My Aunt Bessie, a belly dancer, had breast cancer.

So sorry! Let me tell you about my gall bladder.

Don't worry! You are still desirable, such a pretty face.

My mom looked forward to chemo. She wanted to lose weight!

Don't fret about your husband. I'll take care of him.

What did you do to deserve this?

You don't look sick.

You did want a break. Now everyone will take care of you.

Have a good attitude.

I have an attitude.

SOB

My cancer's name is sob
for every tearful day,
for every angry day.
Son of a Bitch!

Playing the Cancerland Game

Now I'm a blue pawn,
all alone on a rainbow path
filled with peppermint trees,
gumdrop mountains, lollipop landmarks.
Where are all the other pieces?
I avoid Licorice Lagoon, filled with traps
and Bitter Chocolate Bats.
Finally, I arrive at Candy Castle,
live happily ever after.

The game, like cancer:
Cards dealt—surgery, chemo,
radiation, PET scans, MRIs, CAT scans,
blood tests, pills, and shots.
Except the sick world has no landmarks,
no stop signs or lights,
no bonbons and jujubes,
no gingerbread bridges,
no GPS directions.

If I find the exit,
I'll live happily ever after.

A dead beetle

lies on its armored shell,
legs and wings curled like wilted petals.
I throw it in the wastebasket,
wonder about death,
how much time I have wasted.

Chant

Sound energy promotes healing.
Whatever I do, I hear the same incantation.
I have cancer. I have cancer. I have cancer.

I can be at the park with my grandchildren.
I have cancer. I have cancer. I have cancer.
I can be watching *Jeopardy!*
I have cancer. I have cancer. I have cancer.
I can be thumping cantaloupes in the grocery store.
I have cancer. I have cancer. I have cancer.
I can be dancing on the pier, watching a pink sunset.
I have cancer. I have cancer. I have cancer.
I can be filing my nails.
I have cancer. I have cancer. I have cancer.
I can be at Bubba's rib restaurant with friends.
I have cancer. I have cancer. I have cancer.
I can be putting on purple eye shadow.
I have cancer. I have cancer. I have cancer.
I can be opening a fortune cookie.
I have cancer. I have cancer. I have cancer.

The mantra not one for healing.

PART II
CHEMOTHERAPY

The only way to make sense out of change
is to plunge into it.
Move with it and join the dance.

—Alan Watts

First Chemo Appointment

The waiting room is stuffed with people,
beige walls, gray chairs, metal surfaces.
A fake Christmas tree lists to one side.
I'm listing toward chemo:
eight weeks or twelve weeks.
If I keep writing furiously,
maybe they won't call my name.
The TV screen in the middle of the room
says, "Stay positive!" while a voice recites
fun facts about eating well.
Doctor credentials float on the bottom:
Harvard, Duke, and Stanford.
All eyes are glued on it
as if winning lottery numbers
were to be announced.
It's quiet like a church.
I am too embarrassed to cry.
My name is called.

Coke Adds Life

We look at each other
in the chemo waiting room,
try to guess our stories.

The graying man in plaid shorts
and tall tube socks shuffles by.
Was he a banker or a hardware clerk?

The mother with her daughter
reads a *Gourmet* magazine.
Who does the cooking?

The hunky Coke man arrives
to fill the machine,
the clinking cans

the only sound in the room.
I think of Coke ads on TV—
happy polar bears, happy people everywhere—

I walk to the machine,
try to open happiness.

Pain Echoes

An aging nurse poked the chemo needle
into a vein in my right hand. The chemicals leaked,

scorched my skin. Two hours
and nine minutes until the next dose

of oxycodone. The pain throbs like a six-inch thorn
stuck in my foot, or as if my hand

were slammed in a car door,
as if a finger sliced on a broken plate.

It is like eating a hot pepper whole.
I can barely brush my teeth, but I still type.

I need to write this story.
I need a port to take in chemo.

What if I lose my hand?

A slow day

in the chemo room—

some men snore,

others talk of fishing.

Women crochet pink booties for babies.

We're a family of blank, skinny faces.

Few smile.

At every chair chemo bags hang in midair like angels

as their cocktails percolate into our ports.

We recline in drab olive green chairs.

I snuggle under my blanket, sleepy with Benadryl,

try to ignore the piercing sounds of empty bags,

incessant like the sound of trucks backing up.

High-Priced Shot

Chemo kills white blood cells.
    Neulasta shots cut the risk of infection.

The day after chemo, a long needle
    injected into my arm. I count ten, nine, eight...

distract myself from the pain.
    Every joint painful, even my teeth hurt.

Try to think of butterflies, daisies
    blowing in the wind, my grandchildren.

I am Wonder Woman,
    my arms and legs puffed out

with phantom sensations,
    except I'm so weak.

The Scream

> He heard a huge endless scream
> course through nature.
> —Edvard Munch, *The Scream*

Neighbors hear me.
The German lady next door wails with me.
The man above me jumps into his shoes,
runs down to help.
On the street, joggers stop.
The roofer slides down his ladder,
knocks on my door.
Two floors up, the woman worries
I'm having a baby.

The boiling scream starts
from my core, rises.
My lips open wide to let loose
shrieks so loud I scare myself.
Wailing blocks out
the agony of being ripped
open and exposed.
Limp and sweating,
now I am a madwoman.

Power Play

Dina's Hair Salon has a separate room
for chemo patients.

Today my hair is buzzed off.
Why wait for it to fall out in clumps?

The beautician spins my chair around
so I cannot see. The shaver sounds

like a killer bee. My husband holds my hand.
Finished, she twirls the chair

toward the mirror, my eyes large
in a honeydew head.

Empowered. the new me.

Acupuncture

At the Buddhist retreat, I hear
tinkling water fountains and ocean music,

see muted colors and soft lighting.
The bed's crisp sheets comfort me.

The needles, 1/40 the size of sewing pins,
stick in parts of my body to relieve

the intense pain in my hand,
burned in a chemo treatment.

For one hour my body relaxes,
but my mind wants to explode,

break the tranquility in this serene place.
I scream as I pull out the needles.

Chemo Babes

When it's winter in Florida,
Northerners bring flu
so patients stay inside
unless they go for a walk,
germs the enemy.

I walk holding my husband's hand.
Low blood pressure could send me spinning to the sidewalk.
I wear a bright orange dress, a sequined beanie,
and big sunglasses.
People wonder who I am. Smoke and mirrors keep my scars
and needle marks hidden. I'm a pretty pincushion.

No one looks like me.
Where are all the chemo babes?
I need a society of traveling beanies.

Chemo Comedy

A day without laughter is a day wasted.
                            —Charlie Chaplin

I need a laughter pill
with good side effects.
Each day at three, *The Steve Harvey Show*
explodes on the airwaves.
I plump my pillow,
try to forget how tired I feel,
to sit up is a struggle,
the pain intense until Vicodin at four.
I want to "Ask Steve"
how to deal with depression.
I want to counsel sad singles to love each day
and celebrate life by dancing
fast and furious.
"The Good News" section motivates me
to reach out to other breast cancer patients.
In "The Way I See It," Steve looks at the world
in a different way.
I will never look at my life in the same way.
As I snuggle under the covers
for my afternoon nap, "Just One More Thing"
leaves a smile on my face.
I found my new thing.

Bald

I look in the mirror,
see a stranger.

I'm a silent Buddhist monk screaming,
a shiny marble head hiding
in the Louvre's Greek Revival section,
a sobbing Gerber baby,
a piece of popcorn waiting to be popped,
a soft-boiled egg,
a Genoa jellyfish,
a billiard ball bumping off dark corners,
a cherub on the ceiling of the Sistine Chapel.

Baldness takes away anonymity,
says I have cancer,
makes me vulnerable,
raw and exposed.

Cat Lady

Crazy with chemo,

    I tell my husband to buy me cats.

        I say "coffee" instead of "juice,"

    put keys in the refrigerator,

think Friday is Saturday,

    brush teeth with Preparation H,

        try to start my car with a house key.

At Target, I bump into people

    like a bowling ball hits pins,

        abandon my cart in aisle 3,

    walk zigzag to my car.

Bald, thought people might stare,
most try to avoid me.
To see me, too sad.

Turning Point

> Many of our fears are tissue-paper thin,
> and a single courageous step would
> carry us clear through them.
>
> —Brendan Behan

When I heard planes
swoosh over my condo,
imagined one hitting my building.
I wanted to blow up everything.

Cancer, a real threat.
I was so scared,
but halfway through chemo,
I found a ticket of hope.

Found out fear is not a sign
of weakness. Overcoming it,
first step for survival. I'm normal,
can make a successful landing.

American Cancer Society Beauty Day

A bag of goodies can make
me beautiful in two hours.

Chanel lipstick makes a smile brighter.
Mary Kay concealer changes worry to smile lines.
Maybelline eyebrow pencils fill in sparse eyebrows.
OPI pink polish covers yellow nails.
A video shows how tied scarves cover
scars of surgery and bald scalps.
Ten minutes in the wig room,
I pick two: a red one to be daring
and a blond one for sexy nights.

All I really wanted to know was how to keep
my eye makeup on when I cry.

Retail Therapy

Every day at nine,
a message beeps
on my computer.
Shop Zulilly
and I do.
Elmo puppets
for my grandchildren,
yellow, orange, green scarves
to cover my bald head,
blue stone rings
to decorate
my chemo hand,
gold necklaces,
black push-up bras
to enhance my breasts.

Click, Buy.
My closet swells.
Parcels land
at my door.
In three months
I saved $300
on 35 items.
Every day
is my birthday.
The outside world
comes to me.

Rejoice

My strength returns
in the middle of chemo,
a dance party on Fifth Avenue every Friday,

a different band on each street corner.
I wear '60s stretch pants with leather fringe
that flaps around black boots,

a yellow sweater and a matching chemo beanie.
I'm ready to dance. Everyone is moving
to "Celebrate." I throw my head back,

wink at the stars, and howl.

In the Buzz

"Cathy's Clip Joint," the sign hangs crooked.
Combs pickle in jars of blue liquid.
Wheeled trays of rollers line up.
Frank Sinatra croons on a boom box.
Gum-chewing, big-haired, big-butt
beauticians clip and prune.

All thoughts blasted out by beehive dryers,
plastic-caped women sit on Saran-wrapped chairs.
Talking like puppets, lips flap.
Their hair shellacked with Aqua Net,
teased into balls of cotton candy,
guaranteed not to move for a week.

Bald, I sit in the waiting area,
hold my curly wig in my lap.
My name is called.
I sit on a plastic chair,
ask for a shorter style,
one guaranteed not to move for a year.

Payback

In my grandson's favorite cartoon, Olivia
stuffs her pig feet into cherry red high heels.

On a cruise last year, the supersized singer
stuffed her "pig feet" into silver shoes.

We laughed at her, called her Olivia.

Now my feet tingle with neuropathy.
My toes feel fat as pig's toes.

My song now:
> *This little piggy went to chemo,*
> *cried wee wee wee all the way home.*

Armpit and Eyebrows

Armpit, I bathed, shaved, and slathered
deodorant on you.
I took you for granted
until 18 nodes had to be excised.
Today you are like cookie dough,
a red slash across you.
Your glands no longer function.
One good thing, you will never sweat again.

Eyebrows, you were once lush,
well-manicured bushes.
Now thin lines of sparse hairs,
a brown pencil fills in spaces.
Rushing to the gym, I forgot to draw you.
Hours later I looked in the mirror,
both eyebrows half moons.
No one told me.

I sleep alone

always on my right side
on the left side of the bed,
never on my stomach
or left side, my neck too painful
to pivot, my ear numb every morning.
I might need to wear earmuffs for comfort.
My armpit throbs from the removal
of 18 nodes. My left breast burns.

I sleep alone.

I know my husband is in the bed.
I can't see him. I hear him snore lightly,
feel the mattress move when he turns.
When he spoons me, his hand falls asleep.
We are more like knives.
I stare out at a white wall,
a chest of drawers shut tight.

I sleep alone.

The old lady plays piano

every day in the condo above me.
Songs that make me remember:

Dancing in a storm on a rocking cruise ship,
tossed around like a rag doll.

Dancing in LA's hottest nightclub
until the sun woke me up in my neon yellow Pinto.

Dancing with Ingrid, making a sandwich
with a willing man in Las Vegas.

Belly dancing in Istanbul on a stage,
watching the dervishes, my feet whirling.

Dancing at the Holiday Inn where I met
my husband, who proposed three days later.

I'm dancing now in my living room,
out of breath and glorious.

First Night Out

Purple eye shadow, rose lips, dewy face,
legs shining with oil,
a tight blue dress,
bright pink flowers in strategic places:
two on my breasts,
one large blossom on my fertile garden,
strappy heels encircle ankles.

I'm following my mother's advice—diversion.
No one notices my big blond wig
perched on my head.

Last Chemo Appointment

Twelve weeks of misery over,
the nurse ropes pink beads
around my neck,
giving the event a Mardi Gras feel.
The strand like a rosary,
each bead another day of hope.
I stroke the crystals
to foretell my future,
free of cancer.

The room festive like a party,
the IV stand my dance partner,
drip, drip, drip,
beep, beep, beep, a hip-hop song.
Today could be the first day of summer,
my first kiss, my first wedding.
It's like seeing the first star, welcoming a newborn,
hearing the first song that plays on the radio
as once again I get up to dance.

Port Removal Day

Chemo over,
surgery waiting room
the temperature of a meat locker.

LED lights laser down,
like hot spotlights,
the doctor late as usual.

I won't miss you, port,
a button inserted under my skin
to deliver chemo.

The first time a nurse
tried to use it for chemo,
it let me down, no blood.

I ran out of the clinic, yelled,
I'll take three years to live. Screw this!
I don't care.

A concerned nurse grabbed me,
trapped me in a chair,
the next three times success.

I won't miss you, port.
I'm sailing away.

PART III
RADIATION

Dance, when you're broken open.
Dance, if you've torn the bandage off.
Dance, in the middle of fighting.
Dance, in your blood.
Dance, when you're perfectly free.

—Rumi

Ink Art

I'm growing smaller.
Illness takes a little
piece of me every day.

Tattoo time today,
four marks on my skin
to outline the treatment field. Ouch!

The office silent,
I am jumping out
of my seat. My bag of candy bars,

Kindle, and Kleenex falls.
I listen to Flo Rida on my iPod
to calm my crazies.

I'm wearing my Funkadelic T-shirt,
the one I bought at an open mic in NYC,
remember reading my funny poems.

The city alive, everyone going somewhere.
Eight in the room now, everyone alone.
No one going anywhere.

Coming out of the Cocoon

Survived chemotherapy,
time to leave the house.

Don't need its protective
germ-free shell. But I'm no longer

the daring blonde who danced all night
to Rihanna. I'm bald with visible scars,

an X on my breast. I'm not Superwoman
anymore with a pink cape. I'm made of string,

not steel. I'm scared what my friends
will think of me as I crawl out to see.

First Radiation Treatment

It's April Fool's Day.
The joke's on me.
I'm in the Women's Gowned Waiting Room,
leafing through an issue of *Vogue*.
The cover reads "Working It!",
the irony not lost on me.
I slip into the magazine,
become the long-haired beauty
with pouty lips,
feathers around my neck,
dressed in a blue bohemian dress.

It's cold. The radiation rat
lurks in the corner. A serious
nurse comes to get me.
I lie on a skinny bed.
Don't move a muscle, a tech says.
For ten minutes a day, a monster
machine passes over me.
I think of Brian and Martha,
my childhood friends, and old boyfriends:
Tommy, the boy I married in second grade,
Ken, the first boy to get to second base with me.
Only 32 treatments to go,
my nose itches.

What Will My Grandboys Think?

I'm worried as I haven't seen "the boys"
since before chemo. On FaceTime
I wear big hats and colorful turbans.

I'm bald. It's time to show them the real me.
Will they run away screaming?
Will they be frightened?

What will I say to a two-year-old and a five-year-old?
Should I say a ninja shaved my head
or tell the truth?

I say, *Granny is very sick,*
but she'll be fine.

Scent

A spray, a splash
        like a bouquet of a thousand flowers.

Feel feminine. I'm vain.
        Remember my healthy, beautiful self.

The mist, a veil obscuring
        my beat-up body.

Invisible for a moment,
        I'm a woman again,

the most alluring woman in the room.

"Girl" Friends

> Friendship is born at the moment when
> one person says to another, "What? You too?
> I thought I was the only one."
>
> —C. S. Lewis

A circle of short hair, no hair, wigs,
sisters for a few hours.
The topic today areola nipple tattooing—
pictures displayed of breasts
that look like hamburger buns.
The "breast" specialist talks about women
recapturing our former selves.
Promises the tattooing will not
look like two slices of pepperoni.
She wants to be our "cancierge."
She has other services available—
brow tattooing and Voluminizer hair pieces,
permanent makeup—lip color, eyeliner, eyelashes
to make our beauty everlasting.
She drones on, *Self-esteem and self-image so important.*
You can look even better than you did.
Some of us frown, others' eyes tear up.
Some slump in their seats.
We're more than simply beautiful.

We are business owners,
mothers,
pianists,
secretaries,
authors,
wives,

warriors.

Even Rocks Crack

My husband knows how cars,
    electric heaters and toilets work.
Any question, an answer.
    Gramps, why does my snowman melt?
The dahlias in his garden as big as my face.
    A shopping maven, he picks out sexy
dancing dresses for me. Women want to adopt him.
    He loves me,
asked to marry me in three days.
    We danced, traveled, laughed across Europe.

Now cancer.

My husband picks up Percocet and Valium
    and researches the best treatments for me.
Vegetables, fruit, and fish crowd the kitchen. He cooks.
    At chemo appointments, he holds me,
drives me to radiation appointments, blood tests, and scans.
    When I walk he holds my arm as I list to the left.
He orders Raquel Welch wigs and handmade chemo beanies
    to help me look and feel better, invites friends over,
tells long-distance relatives how I am doing,
    leaves funny cards next to my bed.

One day he yelled at the world,
    then took a three-hour drive.

Rainbow Fantasy

I look up at the eight panels
on the ceiling. Silverbells, ambulance white

bloodroot, and pale pink larkspur snuggle
around the green mangrove and white

blackthorn trees. The cobalt blue pond
sparkles under the azure sky.

I picture myself on a purple raft
in a hot pink bikini, tan skin

glistening, long yellow hair
ruffled by a tangerine breeze. A bowl

of sweet red cherries balances on my flat
stomach. An atomic green daiquiri radiates

in one hand. Reality. I'm on a skinny battleship
gray metal bed. The monster arm of the radiation

machine passes over me many times,
like the sun burning through the clouds.

Spud Scraping

At the kitchen sink,
peeler in hand,

I peel potatoes for a family dinner.
Haven't cooked in months,

I'm tired. My back aches.
It's so hard to stand this long.

I dig out the eyes
as they stare at me,

think of them as tumors
in soft flesh,

envision a body free of disease.
My cold hands, numb.

I keep peeling.

To My Friends

You send get-well wishes, funny colorful
cards, inspiring meditation books, oil paints
and canvas, soft blankets for chemo, scented

candles, Godiva chocolates, cheesy casseroles,
brownie treats. Your emails encourage me to stay positive.
Your texts tell me you are thinking of me.

Your phone calls fill me in on gossip. Your visits help me see
there is a world out there. In the middle of the night,
when I am anxious and in despair, I think of you.

Your concern is a light at the end of depression.
Yes, I go through chemo and radiation myself,
but when I think I am alone, your faces appear.

I Really Didn't

I really didn't go into your church.

I really didn't make the Sign of the Cross
with holy water to anoint myself.

I really didn't kneel down on broken knees.

I really didn't light candles to vanquish my darkness—
        the mutilation of my breast,
        the poison in my body,
        the radiation killing my dangerous cells.

I really didn't cry out the Stations,
carrying the heavy cross against my breast.

Day 22

Before the daily "roast,"
we meet in the Gowned Waiting Room:
a Guatemalan, a Romanian, two
African Americans, and a German, me.

In our skins of different colors, we exchange
stories of burns, discuss how MooGoo cream
is the best. We complain about how hard
it is to lie still on the bed for ten minutes.

We share selfies of our former selves,
brag about a grandchild who earned
a yellow belt in tae kwon do.
We bet on who will win *Dancing with the Stars*.

We discuss eating better: Guatemalan tamales colorados,
Romanian cabbage rolls and baked pumpkin,
African-American soul dishes—okra, hog maw—
German red cabbage and rouladen.

With our wigs, scarves and hats,
we smile and laugh though we are frail and tired.
We hold each other in a group hug,
like a family at a reunion.

Dear Muse,

Your cloak of pink, purple,
and yellow feathers masks
my pain and fear.

One day of freedom:
the radiologist says
I am cancer free.

The next day the oncologist
wants a PET scan
after a suspicious blood test.

My throat constricts.
I want to yell,
but for five days I am silent.

Help me, Muse.
Write these words on paper.
This time cancer has taken my voice.

Speechless,
Janay

Climbing Backward

It's April.
An old poinsettia sits
in the corner
of the PET scan waiting room.
Half the leaves
are missing,
the color a fading red.
I feel like the plant,
pale and fragile,
climb inside myself.
Will I be alive
next Christmas?
My iPod plays
Pitbull's "Rain Over Me."
I want to dance, scream,
punch out the air.
Poof!
I evaporate in a cloud
of pink dust,
return to ashes.

If I don't make it
to next Christmas,
pour me into an urn
and put me on the mantel.

A Long Drink

A sad woman
swallowed a miserable monster,
plucked from her back that miserable monster.

A sad woman
swallowed a scary diagnosis.
It slipped and slithered down
to her gizzard.
She swallowed the scary diagnosis
to catch the miserable monster,
plucked from her back that miserable monster.

A sad woman
swallowed the horrors of surgery, chemo, and radiation.
They tasted bitter and rancid.
She swallowed the horrors of surgery, chemo, and radiation
to catch the scary diagnosis.
She swallowed the scary diagnosis
to catch the miserable monster,
plucked from her back that miserable monster.

A sad woman
swallowed her tears.
They made a salty puddle.
She swallowed her tears
to catch the scary diagnosis,
to catch the horrors of surgery, chemo, and radiation.
She swallowed her tears
to catch the miserable monster,
plucked from her back that miserable monster.

A sad woman
swallowed a miserable monster,
a scary diagnosis,
the horrors of surgery, chemo, and radiation,
her tears.
Why did she feel so empty?

The Price

My bones ache from hormone-suppression pills.
My knees, with faces like old ladies, hurt.

In the night, legs move like windmill blades.
Gasping, I hope for a second wind.

Morning I wake with hands like claws,
feet fat with neuropathy. Hot flashes

drench my clothes. I keep fans on high. I am a wild
woman. No matter how much I rest, I'm still tired.

My mind swirls in a tornado.
My safe house of sanity blows away.

I'm a lost Dorothy. If I click my heels,
will I be home again?

Lite Cancer

A "friend" said I was lucky. My cancer wasn't too bad.
I had a lumpectomy, not a mastectomy,
18 nodes excised under my arm, only one cancerous,
three months of chemo, not six, TC the least toxic,
only 33 radiation treatments,
stage 2A, not 4, no recurrence so far.
Retired, I didn't work,
my children grown and gone.
My husband prepared my meals,
picked up my prescriptions,
chauffeured me to doctor appointments.

I had cancer.
Hell, I went through Hell.

Last Day of Radiation

While I lie on the bed for the last time,

I visualize a pink ribbon passing through my heart,

down my throat. It connects to the top of my head

and gives me peace. The ribbon continues skyward,

touches a star, and hangs on the moon.

I breathe deeply.

Another ribbon hooks to my heart,

cascades to my knees, loops around my toes.

I feel calm.

The ribbon tethers me to the ground.

I find joy and relief.

Breast Cancer Survey

Multiple Choice (Circle One)
I am
a. bald.
b. scarred.
c. angry.
d. a Goddess.
e. a Survivor.
f. all of the above.
g. none of the above.

Doctors
a. spend 15 minutes with each patient.
b. order every test known.
c. don't know their patients.
d. recite this mantra: When in doubt, cut it out.
e. say, *We have a situation here.*
f. all of the above.
g. none of the above.

Breast cancer patients
a. yearn for doctors' attention.
b. are frightened.
c. hate pink.
d. are lymphomaniacs.
e. hate Hooters.
f. all of the above.
g. none of the above.

Rank in Order of Importance
___ feel better
___ get better
___ vent better

Post-Treatment Depression

Each week at 10:20, I lie
on the radiation bed for ten minutes,
33 days, boring, but necessary.

I fantasize about day 34,
the freedom of no doctors,
tests, infusions, procedures.

My normal so long has been illness.
Day 34 I am blue,
miss the sick world, the routine.

I realize how the blanket of treatment
protected me. Like a kaleidoscope,
with every new twist, a pattern of new loss appears.

What will my "new normal" be?

PART IV
THE NEW NORMAL

The journey in between what you once were
and who you are now becoming
is where the dance of life really takes place.
                                    —Barbara de Angelis

After cancer I
am worn out, strung out, cried out,
boneless unattached

Transition

Once my yellow hair fluttered like a cape when I danced,
thick eyebrows defined my square face,
generous lips puckered with a peaked cupid's bow,
dark kohl-lined eyes flirted,
a tight pink dress covered a curvaceous body,
cleavage spilled from a lacy bra,
thigh-high nylons clicked into the hooks of garters,
I tangoed in spiky heels.

Then a building exploded.

Now, bald, hollowed by a surgeon's knife,
bonfires burn in my chest,
lymph nodes numb
when I throw my pipe arms
in the dancing air,
a constellation of ragged red scars
on my breast and under my arm.
A port scar sails under my tank top strap.
Down-speckled legs pole down.

I tunnel into my ruined self
and transition to a scarred warrior.

Walls Close In

Coming home to my condo in Florida
after recuperating in New York, the horizon ends

in ice cream clouds topped with thunderheads.
Important doctor checkups still loom.

I open the front door. My chemo blanket
is folded neatly on a chair, an indentation

on my couch where I sat for hours watching the
Lifetime channel. Wigs and chemo beanies jam

a crowded closet shelf. A lone roller waits for bangs.
A miniature Superwoman blows a kiss.

Pink beads hang on the bedpost,
sad memories of my "prison."

I put the condo on the market.

Pink October

Flick on *Good Morning America,*
Breast Cancer Awareness Month,
pink dresses and pompoms swirl on the screen.
I hope for a good morning,
first mammogram since surgery—
my teeth grind, my stomach makes a somersault,
my head pulses with a migraine from conflicting thoughts:
You're fine. You have more cancer.

I crawl into the airless car. Listen to "Monster Mash"
as my deceased brother dances into my head. The office,
cold like my numb hands. "Ain't No Mountain High Enough"
hangs on a sign in the x-ray room.

Hold my breath and freeze.
Hold my breath and freeze.
Hold my breath and freeze.

Breathe.

Delicate

I ate nine York Peppermint Patties
when I was ten. My stomach feels
like that now on my way
to a new oncologist.

Breathless, I climb two flights.
The office standard wood chairs
and a Keurig coffeemaker.
A sad plant in the corner

once an orchid blossom,
now has wood sticks tied to its bare tendrils.
I am like a hothouse flower,
needing so much care—

medicine, doctors, scans,
physical and emotional support—
to hold me up
until I can bloom again.

A Second Opinion

My new oncologist tells me I did not need chemo last year. My onca score 14, rate of cancer recurrence so low chemo would have no effect. Third oncologist agreed. Now the aftereffects— the chemo in my brain, the tingling in my toes, the numbness in my hand.

My mind is still a sandstorm obliterating all my reason. Three months of bone pain, tiredness, anxiety, depression, baldness. Angry, I want to shake my doctor like a rattle. I want to cry out three questions: Did she want to make more money pushing chemo? Did she understand how I would suffer? Did she care?

Bitch-Slap a Woman at Walmart

I needed to buy blush for my pallid face,
but the aisle is too small for two carts.
Could you move your cart please? I ask her.

The woman looks past me, ignores me.
I feel like a firecracker ready to go off.
I want to yell, *See me!* I want to slap her.

Anger, always just below the surface,
hides my fears.
I'm sweet one moment, Godzilla the next.

I need safe ways to express my fury—
    beat up a pillow
    smash a plate
    eat a carton of ice cream

Now I stop. This woman isn't worth it.
I picture my husband being summoned on the loudspeaker.
My cheeks are pink now. I no longer need makeup.
I back away.

Advanced Hindsight

If only I
    had a mammogram yearly.
    didn't smoke or drink.
    ate less sugar.
    exercised and lost weight.
    didn't take estrogen pills back then.

But the present is now.

Self-control requires self-control.
Regret and guilt can't change anything.
Any day could be a recurrence.

I'm ready now,
no flight—fight.

My Husband

A veteran of the breast cancer war,

grows a beard and mustache,

gains twenty pounds.

He's arming himself for the next battle.

I look different too,

short gray and silver hair,

ten pounds lost.

Scars cover my body.

We disguise ourselves.

We hide.

If there's another war,

we are going AWOL.

I worry

when my hip hurts,
it's just a bruise from banging into a drawer.
When my stomach rumbles in pain,
it's just an overly rich dinner.
When my skin looks sallow,
it's just the sun hasn't shone for days.
When my shoulder hurts,
it's just my purse is loaded down with junk.
When I lose my balance,
it's just I'm dizzy from not eating.
When I feel exhausted,
it's just I've been biking too much.
When my breast burns,
it's just from digging out tulip bulbs.
When my back aches,
it's just from lifting too many shopping bags.

Always on alert for the Grim Reaper
making my tumor markers rise
before my shoes dig under.

Touch

may i touch said he

—e. e. cummings

You are so beautiful,
my husband moans.
No hair and scarred,
he loves my blond wig,
colorful scarves and beanies,
thinks I look sexy.

Candles flicker with memories.
He looks at me like he did
when he met me.
Our arms and legs intertwine,
an erotic dance.

Tentatively he touches my scars,
the bedsheets damp. Marvin Gaye's
song "Sexual Healing" plays in my head.
So much in love,
my eyes water.

Online Reading

I google Arimidex, my hormone-suppression drug.
Read about weight gain, feel my stomach bloat.

Read about hair thinning and hair loss, buy Rogaine.
Read about nausea, feel my stomach churn.

Read about hot flashes, buy nightgowns
that wick the sweat.

Read about depression,
count my blessings that I am alive.

Read about breast cancer survivors
full of endless debilitating pain, feel sad.

Read about remission and recurrence,
buy a cemetery plot.

A Secret under My Clothes

Strangers see penciled eyebrows, a crew cut,
a flowing dress a stone necklace, leather bracelets.

Some think I'm a hipster,
edgy and effortlessly cool.

Some think I'm a tree-kissing vegan who wears
natural-fiber clothes, hoop earrings, and Birkenstocks.

Some think I'm a lesbian,
smile, and try to hit on me.

I am a mystery to all.
Only I know the truth.

I am a survivor.

A Bout of Depression

I step into the boxing ring
with my sparring partner, Arimidex,
who tries to suppress my hormones.

She raises her arm, yells,
I will make you weak and depressed.
I feel myself backpedaling, crawling into myself,

too tired to bob and weave or go the distance.
I'm annoyed with her, teary eyed, and in an "empty mood."
Anxiety tickles its way up my neck like a centipede.

I'm her punching bag in a slugfest.
I've decided to stay with her for five years,
the final blow.

I'm down and out,
but I know she is survival.
I hate her.

I need her.

Manikin Head Mandy

She was the prettier me. When I ranted,
she listened, never interrupted me, a great friend
through chemo and radiation treatments.
I wore her blond hair, curly and straight,
looked glamorous, but we both
knew it was an illusion.

She's abandoned in the corner
of my bedroom. What is she thinking?
Now Mandy stares each morning,
dreamy expression, bright pink lips and
flawless complexion, her eyes gray
like mine, dark eyelashes
and thick eyebrows, a stork neck.

Sometimes now I hear her whisper,
Eat right, exercise, and dance.
Today my own hair is two inches long.
Her hair blows around her face.
It's all hers now,
time to let her go.

Don't Sweat the Small Stuff

The line at Rite Aid is so long.
White-haired ladies open their purses,
pull out coupons, and slowly count their coins.

Children scream like sirens,
grab M&M's and bubble gum.
The cashier, befuddled, screws up someone's change.

I am in the middle of the line
waiting to pick up my hormone-suppression pills.
Normally I would be annoyed and angry,

but I had breast cancer.
My mind wanders, pictures purple-tailed mermaids
in calm blue waters.

Damaged Goods

My breast betrayed me with illness.
Surgery maimed me.
A year after I still can't look in the mirror
to see my dented misshapen pear.
I want to remember myself as I was,
curvaceous and full bosomed.
All my parts work, but I feel damaged.

But in my mind today,
I unzip myself like a sleeping bag,
look in my inner mirror, reflect on my stuffing.
My heart beats with love for family and friends.
I feel thankful for a new philosophy.
I get the big picture.
I don't focus on the small stuff.
I take an oath to never stop dancing.
I step into my power, reclaim myself.

Tonight I'm going braless.

Beginning Again

My body is weary,

but a familiar old emotion surges

through me from the top

of my head to the bottom

of my heels. I feel my feet firmly

planted in the earth.

Roots hold me upright and tall.

My head high, I shout,

I'm alive. My shoes start

to dance again to the rhythm of life.

Come dance with me.

ACKNOWLEDGMENTS

I did not take this journey alone. My thanks to...

everyone at the Writers' Center at Chautauqua, the Naples Poetry Group, and the Naples Writers' Forum for their encouragement and critiques; Joan Murray, for all her special editing help; and especially to all the poets who wrote such wonderful endorsements

my first readers—Mari Messer, Gail Lester, Carol Wilke, Jan Tramontano, Carol Townsend, Carol Collins, George Mathon, and Dr. Khalid Rehman—and my editor, Amy Hollis, without whose help this book would never have been published

my children, Jim and Teddie, and their spouses, Kim and Pat, who were with me every step of the way

my grandchildren, Pat Jr. and Teddy, who never looked at me differently and who love me with the pure love of children

my friends, who showed me true friendship with their calls, cards, and gifts

my husband, Richard, whom I can never thank enough for his emotional and physical support

ABOUT THE AUTHOR

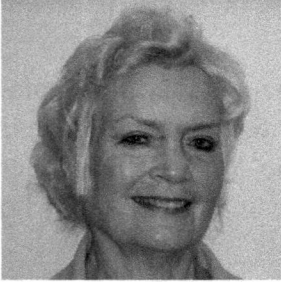

Janay Cosner is a fun-loving poet. She is also a former English teacher and the author of eight Formula Writing curriculum guides for grades K–12.

Even though breast cancer ran in her family, she was shocked and overwhelmed when she was diagnosed with stage 2A. She was always the first one on the dance floor until her dance partner became cancer. Her cancer dance spun her in circles, and she became weak. Her only dance then was a dance with words—poetry.

Writing poems helped her vent and get through doctors' appointments, surgeries, night blues, and long days. Each poem is a snapshot of her journey.

She now rocks a new, beautiful dance of life with her husband in Florida and New York.

9 780692 855553